21-DAY LOG BOOK FOR ACHIEVING WELLNESS GOALS

NCWC's Nutrition 101 Series

A. Sehatti, RN, MSN
Family Nurse Practitioner

NCWC/Amend-Health Press

21-DAY LOG BOOK FOR ACHIEVING WELLNESS GOALS. *NCWC'S NUTRITION 101 SERIES.* Copyright © 2021 by A. Sehatti, RN, MSN, Family Nurse Practitioner.

ISBN 978-0-578-90920-2 (paperback)

Self-monitoring tool   Weight Management   Lifestyle Changes

Printed and bounded in the United States of America
First Printing March 2021

Published by:
NCWC/Amend-Health Press
AKA Nutritional Counseling and Weight Control Clinic
51 E. Campbell Avenue, Suite 129 - 154
Campbell, CA 95008
United States
www.NCWC-AmendHealthPress.com
www.EatActThinkHealthy.com

About the Author

A. Sehatti is a registered nurse and family nurse practitioner. She received her bachelor's degree in nursing from University of Pennsylvania and her master's degree in nursing from University of California, Los Angeles. Aside from her clinical work at such places as Caltech Health Center, UCLA, and Stanford Medical Center, she has over forty years of experience in educating adults and children on weight management, nutrition, and total wellness. A. Sehatti is highly dedicated to making a difference in people's lives. She currently works as a nutritional consultant and health educator at a private practice that she established in 2005 in Northern California. It has been the reward of witnessing people reach their health and wellness goals that has inspired her to write her books and share the tools that have helped her clients with her readers.

Books Published by A. Sehatti

BUILDING A STRONG SENSE OF SELF
Embarking on the Journey of Change
The Inner Control Is the True Control - Book 1

ACCOUNTABILITY AND EMPOWERMENT
A Four-Step Strategy for Overcoming Resentment
The Inner Control Is the True Control - Book 2

THE INNER CONTROL IS THE TRUE CONTROL
WORKBOOK, SECOND EDITION
Inspirational Scripts

A TOOL FOR LETTING GO OF RESENTMENT AND ANGER
Short. Straightforward. Transformative.

A WORKBOOK FOR OVERCOMING RESENTMENT
Mindfulness Scripts

A HANDBOOK FOR DEALING WITH SUGAR
CRAVINGS AND DEPENDENCY
NCWC's Nutrition 101 Series

NCWC'S NUTRITION 101 WORKBOOK
NCWC's Nutrition 101 Series

21-DAY LOG BOOK FOR ACHIEVING WELLNESS GOALS provides you with charts to easily record and track your daily food intake, activity, and behavior for twenty-one days. Doing so will enable you to stick to your plans and build healthy habits.

This helpful logbook also provides you with weekly progress charts. Monitoring and evaluating your dietary, activity, and behavioral patterns will enable you to become aware and identify the areas that you need to work on in order to achieve your goals.

The clinically-proven techniques used in this logbook are designed and organized according to the nutrition education curriculum offered by A. Sehatti, RN, FNP at Nutritional Counseling and Weight Control Clinic.

YOUR DAILY DIET GOAL

FOOD GROUPS	NUMBER OF SERVINGS				
	Break-fast	Snack	Lunch	Snack	Dinner
Grains 1 Serving = 80 Calories					
Starchy Vegetables and Legumes 1 Serving = 80 Calories					
Vegetables: Raw and Cooked 1 Serving = 25 Calories *(1 cup raw or 1/2 cup cooked)*					
Fruits 1 Serving = 60 Calories					
Dairy (1 Serving = 90-120 Calories)					
Meats and Meat substitutes (1 Serving = Varies)					
Fats (1 Serving = 45 Calories)					

YOUR DAILY PHYSICAL ACTIVITY GOAL(S)

TYPE(S)	DURATION

YOUR DAILY BEHAVIORAL MODIFICATION GOAL(S)

1.
2.
3.

COMMENTS

DAY 1 FOOD LOG

TIME	FOOD	AMOUNT	CALORIES	COMMENTS (e.g., Cravings, Symptoms, Feelings)
6-11 AM				
11-4 PM				
4-8 PM				
8-6 AM				

COMMENTS

DAY 1 SELF-EVALUATION

YOUR FOOD INTAKE FOR THE DAY	Fruit	Raw Veggie	Complete Protein (All 3 Meals)	Whole Grain, Legume, Starchy Veggie	Dairy	Water	Others
Total Number of Servings Consumed for the Day							

YOU PHYSICAL ACTIVITY FOR THE DAY	DURATION

THE BEHAVIOR MODIFICATION(S) YOU MAINTAINED FOR THE DAY

COMMENTS

DAY 2 FOOD LOG

TIME	FOOD	AMOUNT	CALORIES	COMMENTS (e.g., Cravings, Symptoms, Feelings)
6-11 AM				
11-4 PM				
4-8 PM				
8-6 AM				

COMMENTS

DAY 2 SELF-EVALUATION

YOUR FOOD INTAKE FOR THE DAY	Fruit	Raw Veggie	Complete Protein (All 3 Meals)	Whole Grain, Legume, Starchy Veggie	Dairy	Water	Others
Total Number of Servings Consumed for the Day							

YOU PHYSICAL ACTIVITY FOR THE DAY	DURATION

THE BEHAVIOR MODIFICATION(S) YOU MAINTAINED FOR THE DAY

COMMENTS

DAY 3 FOOD LOG

TIME	FOOD	AMOUNT	CALORIES	COMMENTS (e.g., Cravings, Symptoms, Feelings)
6-11 AM				
11-4 PM				
4-8 PM				
8-6 AM				

COMMENTS

DAY 3 SELF-EVALUATION

YOUR FOOD INTAKE FOR THE DAY	Fruit	Raw Veggie	Complete Protein (All 3 Meals)	Whole Grain, Legume, Starchy Veggie	Dairy	Water	Others
Total Number of Servings Consumed for the Day							

YOU PHYSICAL ACTIVITY FOR THE DAY	DURATION

THE BEHAVIOR MODIFICATION(S) YOU MAINTAINED FOR THE DAY

13

COMMENTS

DAY 4 FOOD LOG

TIME	FOOD	AMOUNT	CALORIES	COMMENTS (e.g., Cravings, Symptoms, Feelings)
6-11 AM				
11-4 PM				
4-8 PM				
8-6 AM				

COMMENTS

DAY 4 SELF-EVALUATION

YOUR FOOD INTAKE FOR THE DAY	Fruit	Raw Veggie	Complete Protein (All 3 Meals)	Whole Grain, Legume, Starchy Veggie	Dairy	Water	Others
Total Number of Servings Consumed for the Day							

YOU PHYSICAL ACTIVITY FOR THE DAY	DURATION

THE BEHAVIOR MODIFICATION(S) YOU MAINTAINED FOR THE DAY

17

COMMENTS

DAY 5 FOOD LOG

TIME	FOOD	AMOUNT	CALORIES	COMMENTS (e.g., Cravings, Symptoms, Feelings)
6-11 AM				
11-4 PM				
4-8 PM				
8-6 AM				

COMMENTS

DAY 5 SELF-EVALUATION

YOUR FOOD INTAKE FOR THE DAY	Fruit	Raw Veggie	Complete Protein (All 3 Meals)	Whole Grain, Legume, Starchy Veggie	Dairy	Water	Others
Total Number of Servings Consumed for the Day							

YOU PHYSICAL ACTIVITY FOR THE DAY	DURATION

THE BEHAVIOR MODIFICATION(S) YOU MAINTAINED FOR THE DAY

COMMENTS

DAY 6 FOOD LOG

TIME	FOOD	AMOUNT	CALORIES	COMMENTS (e.g., Cravings, Symptoms, Feelings)
6-11 AM				
11-4 PM				
4-8 PM				
8-6 AM				

COMMENTS

DAY 6 SELF-EVALUATION

YOUR FOOD INTAKE FOR THE DAY	Fruit	Raw Veggie	Complete Protein (All 3 Meals)	Whole Grain, Legume, Starchy Veggie	Dairy	Water	Others
Total Number of Servings Consumed for the Day							

YOU PHYSICAL ACTIVITY FOR THE DAY	DURATION

THE BEHAVIOR MODIFICATION(S) YOU MAINTAINED FOR THE DAY

COMMENTS

DAY 7 FOOD LOG

TIME	FOOD	AMOUNT	CALORIES	COMMENTS (e.g., Cravings, Symptoms, Feelings)
6-11 AM				
11-4 PM				
4-8 PM				
8-6 AM				

COMMENTS

DAY 7 SELF-EVALUATION

YOUR FOOD INTAKE FOR THE DAY	Fruit	Raw Veggie	Complete Protein (All 3 Meals)	Whole Grain, Legume, Starchy Veggie	Dairy	Water	Others
Total Number of Servings Consumed for the Day							

YOU PHYSICAL ACTIVITY FOR THE DAY	DURATION

THE BEHAVIOR MODIFICATION(S) YOU MAINTAINED FOR THE DAY

COMMENTS

AN OVERVIEW OF WEEK 1

DAYS OF WEEK 1	NUMBER OF SERVINGS						
	Fruit	Raw Veggie	Complete Protein (All 3 Meals)	Whole Grain, Legume, Starchy Veggie	Dairy	Water	Others
DAY 1							
DAY 2							
DAY 3							
DAY 4							
DAY 5							
DAY 6							
DAY 7							

NUMBER OF MINUTES ENGAGED IN AEROBIC ACTIVITY						
DAY 1	DAY 2	DAY 3	DAY 4	DAY 5	DAY 6	DAY 7

BEHAVIOR MODIFICATION GOAL(S) ACHIEVED						
DAY 1	DAY 2	DAY 3	DAY 4	DAY 5	DAY 6	DAY 7
☐ YES ☐ NO	☐ YES ☐ NO	☐ YES ☐ NO	☐ YES ☐ NO	☐ YES ☐ NO	☐ YES ☐ NO	☐ YES ☐ NO

NEW LEARNINGS

DAY 8 FOOD LOG

TIME	FOOD	AMOUNT	CALORIES	COMMENTS (e.g., Cravings, Symptoms, Feelings)
6-11 AM				
11-4 PM				
4-8 PM				
8-6 AM				

COMMENTS

DAY 8 SELF-EVALUATION

YOUR FOOD INTAKE FOR THE DAY	Fruit	Raw Veggie	Complete Protein (All 3 Meals)	Whole Grain, Legume, Starchy Veggie	Dairy	Water	Others
Total Number of Servings Consumed for the Day							

YOU PHYSICAL ACTIVITY FOR THE DAY	DURATION

THE BEHAVIOR MODIFICATION(S) YOU MAINTAINED FOR THE DAY

COMMENTS

DAY 9 FOOD LOG

TIME	FOOD	AMOUNT	CALORIES	COMMENTS (e.g., Cravings, Symptoms, Feelings)
6-11 AM				
11-4 PM				
4-8 PM				
8-6 AM				

COMMENTS

DAY 9 SELF-EVALUATION

YOUR FOOD INTAKE FOR THE DAY	Fruit	Raw Veggie	Complete Protein (All 3 Meals)	Whole Grain, Legume, Starchy Veggie	Dairy	Water	Others
Total Number of Servings Consumed for the Day							

YOU PHYSICAL ACTIVITY FOR THE DAY	DURATION

THE BEHAVIOR MODIFICATION(S) YOU MAINTAINED FOR THE DAY

COMMENTS

DAY 10 FOOD LOG

TIME	FOOD	AMOUNT	CALORIES	COMMENTS (e.g., Cravings, Symptoms, Feelings)
6-11 AM				
11-4 PM				
4-8 PM				
8-6 AM				

COMMENTS

DAY 10 SELF-EVALUATION

YOUR FOOD INTAKE FOR THE DAY	Fruit	Raw Veggie	Complete Protein (All 3 Meals)	Whole Grain, Legume, Starchy Veggie	Dairy	Water	Others
Total Number of Servings Consumed for the Day							

YOU PHYSICAL ACTIVITY FOR THE DAY	DURATION

THE BEHAVIOR MODIFICATION(S) YOU MAINTAINED FOR THE DAY

COMMENTS

DAY 11 FOOD LOG

TIME	FOOD	AMOUNT	CALORIES	COMMENTS (e.g., Cravings, Symptoms, Feelings)
6-11 AM				
11-4 PM				
4-8 PM				
8-6 AM				

COMMENTS

DAY 11 SELF-EVALUATION

YOUR FOOD INTAKE FOR THE DAY	Fruit	Raw Veggie	Complete Protein (All 3 Meals)	Whole Grain, Legume, Starchy Veggie	Dairy	Water	Others
Total Number of Servings Consumed for the Day							

YOU PHYSICAL ACTIVITY FOR THE DAY	DURATION

THE BEHAVIOR MODIFICATION(S) YOU MAINTAINED FOR THE DAY

COMMENTS

DAY 12 FOOD LOG

TIME	FOOD	AMOUNT	CALORIES	COMMENTS (e.g., Cravings, Symptoms, Feelings)
6-11 AM				
11-4 PM				
4-8 PM				
8-6 AM				

COMMENTS

DAY 12 SELF-EVALUATION

YOUR FOOD INTAKE FOR THE DAY	Fruit	Raw Veggie	Complete Protein (All 3 Meals)	Whole Grain, Legume, Starchy Veggie	Dairy	Water	Others
Total Number of Servings Consumed for the Day							

YOU PHYSICAL ACTIVITY FOR THE DAY	DURATION

THE BEHAVIOR MODIFICATION(S) YOU MAINTAINED FOR THE DAY

COMMENTS

DAY 13 FOOD LOG

TIME	FOOD	AMOUNT	CALORIES	COMMENTS (e.g., Cravings, Symptoms, Feelings)
6-11 AM				
11-4 PM				
4-8 PM				
8-6 AM				

COMMENTS

DAY 13 SELF-EVALUATION

YOUR FOOD INTAKE FOR THE DAY	Fruit	Raw Veggie	Complete Protein (All 3 Meals)	Whole Grain, Legume, Starchy Veggie	Dairy	Water	Others
Total Number of Servings Consumed for the Day							

YOU PHYSICAL ACTIVITY FOR THE DAY	DURATION

THE BEHAVIOR MODIFICATION(S) YOU MAINTAINED FOR THE DAY

COMMENTS

DAY 14 FOOD LOG

TIME	FOOD	AMOUNT	CALORIES	COMMENTS (e.g., Cravings, Symptoms, Feelings)
6-11 AM				
11-4 PM				
4-8 PM				
8-6 AM				

COMMENTS

DAY 14 SELF-EVALUATION

YOUR FOOD INTAKE FOR THE DAY	Fruit	Raw Veggie	Complete Protein (All 3 Meals)	Whole Grain, Legume, Starchy Veggie	Dairy	Water	Others
Total Number of Servings Consumed for the Day							

YOU PHYSICAL ACTIVITY FOR THE DAY	DURATION

THE BEHAVIOR MODIFICATION(S) YOU MAINTAINED FOR THE DAY

COMMENTS

AN OVERVIEW OF WEEK 2

DAYS OF WEEK 2	NUMBER OF SERVINGS						
	Fruit	Raw Veggie	Complete Protein (All 3 Meals)	Whole Grain, Legume, Starchy Veggie	Dairy	Water	Others
DAY 1							
DAY 2							
DAY 3							
DAY 4							
DAY 5							
DAY 6							
DAY 7							

NUMBER OF MINUTES ENGAGED IN AEROBIC ACTIVITY						
DAY 1	DAY 2	DAY 3	DAY 4	DAY 5	DAY 6	DAY 7

BEHAVIOR MODIFICATION GOAL(S) ACHIEVED						
DAY 1	DAY 2	DAY 3	DAY 4	DAY 5	DAY 6	DAY 7
☐ YES ☐ NO	☐ YES ☐ NO	☐ YES ☐ NO	☐ YES ☐ NO	☐ YES ☐ NO	☐ YES ☐ NO	☐ YES ☐ NO

NEW LEARNINGS

DAY 15 FOOD LOG

TIME	FOOD	AMOUNT	CALORIES	COMMENTS (e.g., Cravings, Symptoms, Feelings)
6-11 AM				
11-4 PM				
4-8 PM				
8-6 AM				

COMMENTS

DAY 15 SELF-EVALUATION

YOUR FOOD INTAKE FOR THE DAY	Fruit	Raw Veggie	Complete Protein (All 3 Meals)	Whole Grain, Legume, Starchy Veggie	Dairy	Water	Others
Total Number of Servings Consumed for the Day							

YOU PHYSICAL ACTIVITY FOR THE DAY	DURATION

THE BEHAVIOR MODIFICATION(S) YOU MAINTAINED FOR THE DAY

65

COMMENTS

DAY 16 FOOD LOG

TIME	FOOD	AMOUNT	CALORIES	COMMENTS (e.g., Cravings, Symptoms, Feelings)
6-11 AM				
11-4 PM				
4-8 PM				
8-6 AM				

COMMENTS

DAY 16 SELF-EVALUATION

YOUR FOOD INTAKE FOR THE DAY	Fruit	Raw Veggie	Complete Protein (All 3 Meals)	Whole Grain, Legume, Starchy Veggie	Dairy	Water	Others
Total Number of Servings Consumed for the Day							

YOU PHYSICAL ACTIVITY FOR THE DAY	DURATION

THE BEHAVIOR MODIFICATION(S) YOU MAINTAINED FOR THE DAY

COMMENTS

DAY 17 FOOD LOG

TIME	FOOD	AMOUNT	CALORIES	COMMENTS (e.g., Cravings, Symptoms, Feelings)
6-11 AM				
11-4 PM				
4-8 PM				
8-6 AM				

COMMENTS

DAY 17 SELF-EVALUATION

YOUR FOOD INTAKE FOR THE DAY	Fruit	Raw Veggie	Complete Protein (All 3 Meals)	Whole Grain, Legume, Starchy Veggie	Dairy	Water	Others
Total Number of Servings Consumed for the Day							

YOU PHYSICAL ACTIVITY FOR THE DAY	DURATION

THE BEHAVIOR MODIFICATION(S) YOU MAINTAINED FOR THE DAY

COMMENTS

DAY 18 FOOD LOG

TIME	FOOD	AMOUNT	CALORIES	COMMENTS (e.g., Cravings, Symptoms, Feelings)
6-11 AM				
11-4 PM				
4-8 PM				
8-6 AM				

COMMENTS

DAY 18 SELF-EVALUATION

YOUR FOOD INTAKE FOR THE DAY	Fruit	Raw Veggie	Complete Protein (All 3 Meals)	Whole Grain, Legume, Starchy Veggie	Dairy	Water	Others
Total Number of Servings Consumed for the Day							

YOU PHYSICAL ACTIVITY FOR THE DAY	DURATION

THE BEHAVIOR MODIFICATION(S) YOU MAINTAINED FOR THE DAY

COMMENTS

DAY 19 FOOD LOG

TIME	FOOD	AMOUNT	CALORIES	COMMENTS (e.g., Cravings, Symptoms, Feelings)
6-11 AM				
11-4 PM				
4-8 PM				
8-6 AM				

COMMENTS

DAY 19 SELF-EVALUATION

YOUR FOOD INTAKE FOR THE DAY	Fruit	Raw Veggie	Complete Protein (All 3 Meals)	Whole Grain, Legume, Starchy Veggie	Dairy	Water	Others
Total Number of Servings Consumed for the Day							

YOU PHYSICAL ACTIVITY FOR THE DAY	DURATION

THE BEHAVIOR MODIFICATION(S) YOU MAINTAINED FOR THE DAY

COMMENTS

DAY 20 FOOD LOG

TIME	FOOD	AMOUNT	CALORIES	COMMENTS (e.g., Cravings, Symptoms, Feelings)
6-11 AM				
11-4 PM				
4-8 PM				
8-6 AM				

COMMENTS

DAY 20 SELF-EVALUATION

YOUR FOOD INTAKE FOR THE DAY	Fruit	Raw Veggie	Complete Protein (All 3 Meals)	Whole Grain, Legume, Starchy Veggie	Dairy	Water	Others
Total Number of Servings Consumed for the Day							

YOU PHYSICAL ACTIVITY FOR THE DAY	DURATION

THE BEHAVIOR MODIFICATION(S) YOU MAINTAINED FOR THE DAY

COMMENTS

DAY 21 FOOD LOG

TIME	FOOD	AMOUNT	CALORIES	COMMENTS (e.g., Cravings, Symptoms, Feelings)
6-11 AM				
11-4 PM				
4-8 PM				
8-6 AM				

COMMENTS

DAY 21 SELF-EVALUATION

YOUR FOOD INTAKE FOR THE DAY	Fruit	Raw Veggie	Complete Protein (All 3 Meals)	Whole Grain, Legume, Starchy Veggie	Dairy	Water	Others
Total Number of Servings Consumed for the Day							

YOU PHYSICAL ACTIVITY FOR THE DAY	DURATION

THE BEHAVIOR MODIFICATION(S) YOU MAINTAINED FOR THE DAY

COMMENTS

AN OVERVIEW OF WEEK 3

DAYS OF WEEK 3	NUMBER OF SERVINGS						
	Fruit	Raw Veggie	Complete Protein (All 3 Meals)	Whole Grain, Legume, Starchy Veggie	Dairy	Water	Others
DAY 1							
DAY 2							
DAY 3							
DAY 4							
DAY 5							
DAY 6							
DAY 7							

NUMBER OF MINUTES ENGAGED IN AEROBIC ACTIVITY						
DAY 1	DAY 2	DAY 3	DAY 4	DAY 5	DAY 6	DAY 7

BEHAVIOR MODIFICATION GOAL(S) ACHIEVED						
DAY 1	DAY 2	DAY 3	DAY 4	DAY 5	DAY 6	DAY 7
☐ YES ☐ NO	☐ YES ☐ NO	☐ YES ☐ NO	☐ YES ☐ NO	☐ YES ☐ NO	☐ YES ☐ NO	☐ YES ☐ NO

NEW LEARNINGS

Self-awareness and self-accountability
are keys to maintaining healthy lifestyle choices.

www.ingramcontent.com/pod-product-compliance
Lightning Source LLC
Chambersburg PA
CBHW072152020426
42334CB00018B/1966